I Pharmacist

I Pharmacist

GHAYDA ALRASS

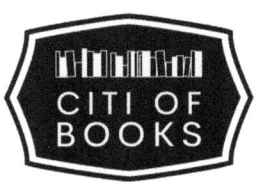

CITI OF BOOKS

CITIOFBOOKS, INC.
3736 Eubank NE Suite A1
Albuquerque, NM 87111-3579
www.citiofbooks.com
Hotline: 1 (877) 389-2759
Fax: 1 (505) 930-7244

Ordering Information:

Quantity sales. Special discounts are available on quantity purchases by corporations, associations, and others. For details, contact the publisher at the address above.

Printed in the United States of America.

ISBN-13:   Softcover   978-1-960952-38-7
                eBook   978-1-960952-39-4

Library of Congress Control Number: 2023910478

TABLE OF CONTENTS

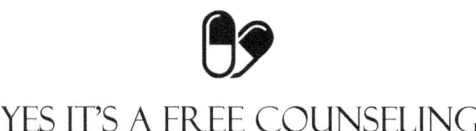

YES IT'S A FREE COUNSELING

So I did my homework, and researched, to answer the question that I keep asking myself: What other profession, besides retail pharmacy, offers and gives free counseling every day to many customers? I did specify "customers," not "patients," because I tried to deal with this subject from the widest possible window—that is, pharmacy as a business and not only a health care provision system.

To be fair, some home stores do offer free consultation for that problem you have in the bathtub, for instance, so that you can try to fix it yourself before you call the specialist. But have you ever called a lawyer for a free consultation or taken your car to the mechanic just to see what the problem is, without paying for the inspection of this problem?

You might think by now that I'm either a money-oriented person or too thrifty when it comes to the time I will spend with this or that patient to answer a question that he or she has when I do not have an obligation to do that!!

Actually, it's neither. (Sorry if I disappointed you.) Our employers want us to provide consultations as a part of our jobs, and we, as health care providers, have known since we went to a pharmacy school that this career is a very special one because it deals with human pain and physical, mental, and emotional needs. Unfortunately, the feedback and the rewards from most patients are very negative, and sometimes this affects our vision of this career in a destructive way.

Here is an example of something that can happen at any retail pharmacy, in any city in our country. A patient calls you and asks about medication. (Keep in mind he is an xy person, for whom you didn't fill any prescription for that specific medication.) Since you have more important responsibilities to take care of in the pharmacy, you probably ask him to hold for a couple of minutes. When you come back to the phone and pick tip line on hold, do you know what is waiting for you? He's raising his voice in an unacceptable manner, complaining about being on hold for longer than two minutes and trying to be sarcastic about your performance (even though he probably doesn't know you at all). You get all of these great emotions from him because you put him on hold, and not because of the way you answered his questions or the content of your answer!

We are, after all, human beings. We have our reactions to everyday life matter, just like any other person in a very different profession and in a completely different situation. So, how can I still be professional, keep my practice, answer the question in a cool manner, and make that person satisfied, if not necessarily happy, with my answer?

I have found only two ways to deal with this situation, and it's up to you which one to choose. First, erase from your mind the first part of the story—the rudeness part—and deal with the caller as if you have just heard a question from a recorder, not a live person. Pretend that, in turn, are answering that recorder. In other words, there is no personal feeling in this scenario. Your second option, since he spoke to you disrespectfully, is to decline to answer the question, politely thank the caller, and hang up the phone.

I always believe in doing what's right, and I believe in kindness as the best thing anybody can give to humanity since it's the easiest, most generous, and the thing we all need in our lives every day. This is especially true in this specific profession, in which people seek help from you. Sometimes, they need somebody to listen more than anything else; their question might appear as a reason behind the call or the contact you get.

Whichever option you chose in this scenario, you do go home with less frustration and more satisfaction with the job. Most importantly, you look forward to the next day as a new day with more challenges in this career.

WHAT IS THE BEST-SELLING HOLIDAY ITEM?

The first things to come to your mind when you think of holidays, like Christmas, for example, are the joy in the atmosphere, the happy spirits for almost everybody, and the special time you spend with family and friends.

Unfortunately, true life experience might tell us otherwise! I have to admit this in two simple words: "I'm surprised." What I'm about to say might not be correct; studies and Gallup polls may show different data regarding the best-selling item during the holidays, when people exchange gifts to show their love and appreciation, and when the consumer's report reported record spending. I said it might not be correct because I didn't do a study that will be in the database of an institute or company or make headlines. I have to admit that I wish somebody would do such a poll so that many people will know this as a fact and maybe even try to change it.

Almost every pharmacy, especially in the retail sector, probably does know this fact, which I tried to make myself think was only a coincidence or happened only to me. But I guess I was wrong.

To make a long story short, I'm talking simply about dispensing anti-anxiety medicine. I see these prescriptions doubled if not tripled, on these occasions. I always thought people were busy finishing their shopping, visiting the mall, and ordering some nice gifts online, but it looks like the community pharmacy and anti-anxiety medicine have priority on many people's lists!

While many people argue with their pharmacists for an early refill of their anti-anxiety medicine, at this time of the year people are more aggressive than at any other time. They seem tense and even panicked. They are not asking simply for a slightly early refill of a prescription for Xanax, Valium, or Ambien, but for very early refills which might reflect overuse of the medication.

We have to admit, whether we like it or not, that our nation is stressed out, and the lifestyles of many people push them down this path. It makes you think: Is there any way out of this? Is it possible to go back in time to three or four decades?

The issues of anxiety, depression, and insomnia are important and wide-open subjects for discussion in our society today. But returning to the main subject, anxiety during the holidays, let's try to put some headlines solutions or at least try to seek some alternatives to the anti-anxiety medication mania at this season of the year.

If the patient who has a perception for anti-anxiety medicine thinks that a one-day holiday during the week or forming a long weekend will make it hard to get that medicine, he or she is wrong, and needs to be told in a more pushy way, it's not the last day we will live our life!

I have found that patients who need this kind of medicine are really putting themselves in a more stressed and panicky situation when they worry more during the holidays about the medicine that they take in the first place to help them with an anxiety disorder. So, it helps for the pharmacist to recommend that these patients slow down and take a deep breath, and enjoy the holidays as much as possible.

The pharmacist can and will play a positive role in dealing with this issue for at least two reasons: First, pharmacists are healthcare providers who are very accessible to the public, and easier to talk to and reach than a doctor (This doesn't mean that they can replace the doctor.) Second, simply because of the shrinking kind of relationships in families, friends, and human beings in general, which make it always nice to find somebody to listen to you and to your problem, at least for the time being, which might give that person some kind of the relief we all needs and look for in our daily human interaction. To be realistic, I can't hope for a completely anxiety-free society, but I can wish for a happy holiday with a lower level of anxiety.

"IS THE WORD 'RESPECT' IN YOUR DICTIONARY?"

I really believe that pharmacy schools should give more attention to, and dedicate longer areas for practice as a retail pharmacist. Even though the subject itself might be mentioned here and there, and some professors might be interested in delivering this kind of information to their students, I believe it should be given more importance in a way that can be helpful for pharmacy students. If they work in the retail sector, they will need at least mental and emotional preparation.

I don't want to be negative in dealing with this subject. Indeed, all I'm trying to say is: "Attention, future pharmacists, it's the hard truth, so be prepared."

One thing I wish for the most is to be able to walk in the patient's (customer's) shoes and use his or her eyes so I will understand how he or she looks at that person who is called a pharmacist.

Since it is not fair to make the case a general one, or a black and white case, then it's more acceptable in my humble opinion today A good percentage of people have the word "respect" in their vocabularies, but they forget it completely when they step inside the pharmacy. The word is absent completely from others' vocabularies. So, the patient who waited for months to see his HMO doctors, or waited while in pain to get a prescription from his MD, came to the pharmacy with complete confidence that since everything he or she wanted is almost clone, it should take only a few minutes to get his medicine and he will be out of this place doing his other, more important business.

And the truth is coming, when the pharmacist says the patient, "Sorry, your prescription is not covered."

At the beginning of this article, I said that pharmacy schools have to prepare their students for retail work. This is one of hundreds of examples of the need to do so.

Here we go—are you ready? (This isn't part of a play on a stage of one infamous show.) The screaming is coining: "What do you mean, it's not covered?"

The pharmacist responds, "Again, sir, you can call the toll-free number for the insurance company; they will be able to explain it to you."

"You don't understand—I'm telling you that I'm covered! I pay them every month, and you come now and say it isn't."

"Of course, we can still call your doctor and ask him for an alternative."

"I don't want any alternative. I like the sample he gave me. Don't try to act on your own and change things the way you like!"

With a faded smile, the pharmacist answers, "Then we can also ask your doctor for something called prior authorization, which is a special request from his office to your insurance company so that the medicine might get covered."

"'Might?' I am losing my patience here, and you stay cool—which proves to me that you don't really care. How long will this prior authorization take?"

"Usually it will take two or three days to get approved."

"Well, I don't think you know what you doing. As a matter of fact, I don't think you know anything. Give me my damn prescription back. And you'd better kiss your job goodbye because I will work on this or you will hear from your employer, I promise you."

Finally, I need to correct myself when I gave the word "respect" all of my attention because I forgot another important one: "Think.". I will be happy if those kinds of patients use either thought or respect. think thinking.

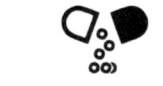

"A FRUSTRATING NIGHT"

The person who helped me that night happened to be a good helper. I guess I was lucky.

You're really lucky when you get a clerk with a problem-solving mentality and a nice customer service attitude. He is just the right person for that exact position in a retail pharmacy.

Since my clerk is a patient person when it comes to customer service, I was surprised to see him lose his patience. He nearly begged me to try to help a customer at the prescription pickup window. "She simply told me, 'I don't think you know what you doing; just get me somebody else.'"

Since I was very busy, and this was the busiest time of the day anyway, I didn't ask him what was going on. I just went ahead to that patient and said the golden sentence in the customer service manual: "Hi, how can I help you?"

According to the patient, her insurance for prescription coverage would end that day. We had filled her prescription for a thirty-day supply of prenatal vitamins, but she wanted to get the advantage and fill a 100-day supply instead. When (began to explain that this issue was up to her insurance company and had nothing to do with our pharmacy, she interrupted me to say, "It's just vitamins."

I tried again to explain that she needed to contact the insurance company, but she couldn't wait for me to finish my sentence to tell me again, "It's just vitamins." At that point, I thought would be only fair to the patient for the pharmacy to perform that service for her, so the pharmacy itself, at the same moment of our discussion (which is almost a discussion from one side) can call the insurance and try to see if they will give the Rx an override for a 100-day supply. I dialed the phone number of the insurance company, and I explained the situation to the agent. He responded exactly as I had done earlier, but I knew that the patient would not believe me unless I let her speak to the insurance agent herself.

As I said, it was a busy night, so after I handed the patient the telephone, I went back to my filling section. I started working on something else, but I could still hear what she was telling that agent. She did spend not less than 7-10 minutes going on and on, repeating the same subject as if she were in a battle with only one possible ending—the three-letter word "Win." After those 7-10 minutes, the patient came back to me. This time, I started the conversation by saying, "So what did he say?" To my surprise, she responded, "It doesn't matter what he said. What really matters is the fact that I have had a lot of problems with your pharmacy lately, and I'm definitely going to take my business somewhere else." So, it was the other night at the pharmacy when the patient approached you with a closed mind, refusing to understand any explanation you try to provide and all you will get at the end is frustration.

"WHAT ABOUT MY RIGHTS?"

Each state's Board of Pharmacy exists to protect the consumer in that particular specific state. Of course, we pharmacists have to pay a certain fee to keep our licenses active. It is a very normal situation that can apply to many different areas in life when it comes to protecting the consumer and the role that any given government office will play it.

The law protects consumers, but who protects us as professionals and human beings when we deal with situations such as inaccurate and invalid accusations by a patient? The story goes like this: A pharmacist received a refill request for a prenatal vitamin. She refilled the prescription.

Then the patient called back to express her anger over this refill case. Why? Because she believed that the pharmacist had filled it incorrectly. The pharmacist checked the patient's profile and found that the prescription was refilled correctly, but it happened that she also had another prescription from a different doctor for a different kind of prenatal vitamin. Since the first rule of customer service is to always try to make him or her happy with the service, the pharmacist didn't hesitate to apologize to the patient for the inconvenience of having to come down to the pharmacy again to pick up her other prenatal vitamins. She didn't forget to remind the patient that it would be really helpful to specify next time which prescription she wanted.

Up to this point, the story is a normal one that can happen anytime. What was abnormal was that the patient came into the pharmacy yelling as much as she can that this incident might have "killed her"!

The pharmacist was already prepared to explain physically to the patient what had really happened by writing a copy of her profile history which showed why this situation had occurred. She apologized to the patient a second time.

The fact of the matter is the patient either believed or acted as if she were convinced that this incident could have killed her. She was acting in a very unacceptable manner, using yelling act, displaying a disrespectful attitude, and harassing and humiliating the pharmacist in front of all the other customers who happened to be standing there.

The pharmacist reacted in a normal way, asking the patient to leave the pharmacy because her behavior was unacceptable and she was disturbing the business.

When you read this scenario, you may think it ended as described above, like many stories which occur in a retail pharmacy on a daily basis. But, unfortunately, that wasn't the end of the story.

Four months from that date, the pharmacist required a little from the state Board of Pharmacy asking for a statement from the dispensing pharmacist, with all the resolved information the patient drugs review and so on.

The first reaction the pharmacist had was how unfair it was that the patient ended up complaining to one of the highest authorities, even though there was no basis for such a complaint.

As I stated above, the state board is basically an agency to protect the consumer; this is fully understandable and completely needed. The only question that forces itself here is: Who protects the pharmacist's rights, especially in a case like this, in which no real mistake occurred? The right as a human being with brain and emotion, with values and ethics, and with all respect to both the law and the consumers!

"DEAR PUBLIC: PHARMACISTS ARE PROFESSIONALS, TOO"

I have to admit that working in a community pharmacy contributed in many ways to my whole view of life and philosophy of dealing with people.

Unfortunately, I still can't understand why the pharmacist as a professional couldn't get much respect, if any, from the public, or at least from those whom he serves and helps every day.

When the California Board of Pharmacy decided to change the law in regard to controlled medicine, which they did in 2004, they didn't really try to educate the three most important people affected by this new regulation: the doctor (the prescriber), the pharmacist (the dispenser) and the patient (the consumer).

I personally think it is, after all, the responsibility of the doctor and the pharmacist to explain these new regulations to the patient.

If the reader has never heard of or come close to this terminology, a quick explanation might help. Controlled medication (medicine that has the potential for dependency, habit formation, and abuse) has been classified into five classes. Class II is the most restricted class in retail pharmacy. When the California Board of Pharmacy decided to make some changes in regard to the types of prescription of controlled medication Class II (Gil), they did not provide enough details. In addition, any process of change will take time, usually regardless in which aspect was that. I think most, if all, pharmacists faced a lot of problems with this issue. One of those cases explains exactly the frustration I have to deal with in this regard.

A patient's mother had been informed by his doctor that this kind of prescription (C-II) is refillable (which has never been the case) and that the new regulation didn't change anything in this area.

When I received a phone call from this mother, after she had already given a hard time to the technician that day, she was already angry and had lost the normal tone of voice that the average person uses in conversation.

I thought the best way to deal with this situation would be to let the person explain herself and make the issue clear for me before I tried to help solve the problem she was facing.

She was very upset about her son's prescription and demanded to know why it had not been refilled yet even after her doctor had said that the regulation allowed this.

After I let her finish, I thought, now my Kali to explain and clarify the whole issue. But I guess she wasn't ready to hear me, since she didn't let me finish my first sentence. Instead, she jumped in and repeated the same story all over again.

I didn't have any choice except to wait for her to calm down so I could say my lines if she allowed me to do so!

When she was out of things to say, I started again by saying, "I, personally, asked a board inspector about this matter, and..."

Again she interrupted me, and this time she iced it with this sentence: "I don't want to listen to you! Just refill it— I don't want to listen to you; can't you understand?"

I think it's impolite to hang up the phone on somebody else, but I did it this time. Not to justify my action, but what else should I have done? I felt so frustrated in a way I can't even describe. Here I was, dealing with somebody who didn't even know any rule of conversation, using unacceptable manners, and asking me to break the law, just because she wanted to and thought it was her right to do so!

After five minutes, I received a complaint from the store manager about that call. I learned that the person had requested my name from him, so that she could lodge a complaint against me with the head office of the company I work for.

Then, ten minutes later, I received a second call from that patient's doctor. I was very clear with her in explaining the new rules on C-II, and that these prescriptions are now refillable. I also gave her all the information I had received from the board inspector, and I didn't forget to explain how frustrated I was with the patient's behavior.

The doctor said that she thought my information was probably correct. So I asked her if she could call the patient and enlighten her about this matter. The doctor assured me that she was ready to go home now, but that she might be able to call her the next day.

"HOLIDAY = AN ANXIOUS, SAD AND PAINFUL TIME."

The issue I will talk about today, I might have mentioned before. I'm really interested in knowing an answer to the question that always surfaces during a holiday or three-day weekend or so.

The first thing to come to your mind regarding holidays is that they are times people have off from work, school, or other obligations. They are also times to spend with family, friends, and loved ones. So, if we don't want to be very optimistic about this subject, at least we'll be expecting a good time you will have on the holiday regardless of what your plan was and how you end up spending the time these days.

I'll try to put my question in a very simple and direct way: Why we are sad, full of anxiety, and completely unhappy during the holidays?

Some statistical studies show that the suicide rate is higher than normal during holiday time, compared to the rest of the year. Since I'm talking about life in a community pharmacy, which means fewer cases of suicide that you might face, my speculation will be mainly about the higher dispensing rate of anti-anxiety, antidepressant, and painkiller medicines.

It is normal and common to learn more about life as you grow older and have more experiences. But I think that I will never, get as much understanding of life, people, and society as I did by working in a community pharmacy. So, since I don't have a scientific study to go by when I'm discussing this matter, I'll rely on a personal experience I had in this area and see if the mystery will be solved so I can resolve my own wonder!

The main area of concern I have is that this time off from work, school and so on gives us more time to think about ourselves.

There is more time to question our own subject of concern, our accomplishments, our relationships, and many other things.

One of the issues that caught my attention is the difference in dispensing rates of these medicines among different ethnic groups.

In my experience in Southern California, this rate is minimal among Hispanic and Asian patients. The only explanation I can think of is that there is more family connection and attachment in these ethnic groups.

After family relationships, comes anxiety. People in our society worry a great deal about the future, especially at the end of a holiday or long weekend. As if this holiday is simply the time we spend worrying about life in the days after the holiday finished. This anxiety basically will take the place of the more enjoyable days we should have during holidays, or at least, normal days if I might say.

Regarding the mystery of increased demands for more pain medicine during these holidays and even during regular weekends, I have to admit, this is the biggest mystery I know, since there is no scientific or medical explanation. There is simply no relationship between holidays and any increase in pain rate or intensity.

The sad conclusion in this regard is that there is a vast emptiness in many people's lives; a hole that must be occupied with something, even if that something will make you drowsy and uncomprehended!

Finally, in discussing this vital issue, I don't intend to be critical. Rather, my intention is focused completely on two things: making our society aware of this problem (and I couldn't use a better way to describe it) and trying to solve it by learning the reasons behind it.

"DO YOU LIKE TO BE THE MESSENGER?"

I guess the word "messenger" can be the equivalent of the pharmacist's job in many ways. Actually, in many cases, the pharmacist might be speechless, and the only word he can say is, "I'm just the messenger."

Of course, this kind of phrase that explains itself will not make many patients happy. Sometimes it can lead to an even worse situation since the patient is in fact forcing this messenger as if he is the sole person with the bad news!

In real life (and forget about all the years you spend in the academic and experimental life of pharmacy school), you will, in fact, deal as the middleman between the patient, his insurance company, and his doctor.

In the case of the insurance company, the patient doesn't really see the insurance agent or read the company's formulary. Basically, all he knows is the amount of his monthly payment to the health insurance company.

Now we come to the practical life when the patient faces the fact that his insurance is not covering the medication the doctor gave him—or it might be covered, but with a very high co-payment.

Unfortunately, these situations occur every clay at any community pharmacy. I always try to put myself in the shoes of patients when they face their problems, but the only thing I wish is for them to try out my shoes! In this way, before anyone could jump on the pharmacist's case, he or she would consider why the pharmacist is not being as helpful as possible, why the co-pay was that much or it costs too much.

Even at that point, the frustration the patient expresses is acceptable to some degree. I give him or her the benefit of the doubt, realizing that he or she might not be aware of the co-payer or the details of the insurance company's formulary.

What is completely unacceptable is turning this frustration into anger, when the fire been shot from one side while the other side is gun-less.

As I mentioned before, every profession requires responsibility toward the party that he provides service to. But at the same time, and in this particular situation, the patient also has some responsibility when it comes to his health insurance coverage.

When the patient is faced with the bitter fact, and this comes through a messenger (the pharmacist), whom do you think it's easier to argue with and get angry at, the insurance agent, whom you don't see, or the pharmacist, who is standing in front of you?

The answer is very easy. So, until the public is well-educated about this matter, would you like to be the messenger?

"HOW IS THE MOOD IN THE TWENTY-FIRST CENTURY?"

Sitting around the table
In a very nice restaurant
Where the decorations are fabulous
And the lighting is relaxing,
The whole setup is ready—
Ready for the hour—
An hour of something.
That something is educational.
The presenter is a doctor.
Excuse me... a specialist doctor.
His area of expertise Is called psychiatric medicine.

I know that stigma
We all had in mind
When we first heard the name
Or even thought for a moment,
He is a psychiatric!
But after meeting this one
I have to say, loudly,
"It's not a stigma.
Rather, it's the truth!"
So don't feel guilty the next time
This idea comes to your mind.

I have to be fair,
Especially in dealing with science—
The science of psychiatry.
The lecture was informative,
And we gained a lot of information.
The presenter didn't forget
To remind us fifteen times
(Fifteen times in a half-hour lecture)
That he is the only psychiatrist in town.

I couldn't wait until he was done.
He allowed us to ask questions or express concerns,
And the surprise was there
When nobody had any concerns.
So I jumped in
To ask the questions of concern.

OK, doctor... it's only one of them
Just a simple answer required
To this important question:
When a child of four years
Is prescribed an antidepressant,
How can he be diagnosed
And the problem was easily solved?

How can you send a kid home
With a bottle to elevate his mood?
How did we forget the diamond quote,
"Diagnose before you prescribe,"
and how you can even diagnose
this illness in a four-year-old?

A hundred-odd years ago
People might have dreamed of a magic world.
The moon was far away.
But the dream was in the mind
And written in many books.
Scientists worked on this thought,
So the dream came true very soon.

Did people in those times
Ever think of the coming century,
In which depression is the main sign
Of the so-called "century twenty-one,"
When kids are given those medications
And even the veterinarian treats your pet
With a dose of antidepressant
Because he thinks that your dog
Is not happy at all....

"WHEN THE FLU VIRUS LAUGHED AT US"

It's not a quiz.
Rather, it's a simple question.
It's something you, or most people,
Get in autumn to prepare for winter.
No, it's no the Christmas gifts.
Nice try, though.
Think more and more.
It's the simple medicine that some of us think—
Truly think and actually believe—
Is the elixir of life.
Time is up. It's the flu shot.

Life is good—at, least that's what we think.
Look at us, with all the success
That mankind has achieved
In technology and etc...
The list is long,
And I don't know how to start
With the human being accomplishments
Just remember where we are:
It's the twenty-first century on Earth.

I'm still surprised
By the whole matter. In fact,
I can't understand the reaction
All those people have
When they hear
There is a shortage of flu shots.

Take it easy, my friend.
I know you were waiting here.
I know you believe in it
And look forward to having it.
 Still, I beg you, please,
To take a moment or a break
And remember it's not a guarantee
That you will never get sick
If this shot given to you
And stays in your system as you want.

For the history record only,
It's sometime in 2004
When the official sources declare
There will be a shortage this year
Because of reasons out of hand
Not everybody will be immunized.
Things can happen sometimes
Against our will and with surprise,
But remember the fact
That it could always be worse.

With all due respect to those in need
Of immediate help and complete check,
I need to say this,
To remind people at large of this:
There is no special magic with this shot.

If you're not completely convinced,
Then go back to the records
To see percentages and numbers
Of people who got sick
Even after injections.
So, the humanity can take a breath
And wake up a little after this mess.

Stand up and laugh your heart out.
It's good to prepare for this reason,
And it's OK if the flu virus plays the game
With a different strategy every year.

The flu viruses laughed at us.
They jumped with manic joy
And said loudly, "I can still play the game,
At least for one more year."
The flu can tell the history and future:
"I was even able to shape the election
when the presidential candidate was asked,
'What happened to the flu shot?'"

"I TRUST YOU—BUT, SORRY, I DON'T RESPECT YOU!"

Whether you are a positive person or a negative one, it's truly rewarding to sit down with only one person—yourself—and look at your life with a clear eye, with no editing. In this way, you will see many decisions that you made, a decision that you can give credit to yourself in it.

My personal belief is that the Lord created each of us to have a unique life, including a sequence of events that's specific to each person. With the above introduction, I have to say that being a pharmacist is one of the greatest things that have happened to me.

If you read the pages preceding this chapter, you might have come to the conclusion that I have a negative attitude toward this profession. But I truly mentally and emotionally love my profession, and I owe the Lord, my parents, and my husband thanks for that.

What made me write about this subject is the question that always pops into my mind, and may have in the minds of many other pharmacists: Why doesn't the public treat the pharmacist with respect?

I beg you to trust me on that because I have honestly tried to find an answer to this question. I love to admit, though, that the answer is not clear!

According to a Gallup poll, pharmacy occupied the number That slot as the most trusted profession between 1990 and 1996. T at is, by itself, an award to make any pharmacist proud and content.

I know that many other pharmacists will agree with me that almost every day at least one patient will mention to his or her Pharmacist, "I trust you more than my physician!"

Regardless of how true or false this statement is, I personally think it is a matter of attention and more time dedicated to the patient than an issue of trust. I say this because I will become a patient someday and I have lived this relationship of patient/doctor thing, which makes me understand what my patients mean by this statement.

I don't like to fool myself or others, so I will not claim that we, as pharmacists, are more trustworthy than doctors. However, I can assure everyone that in general, pharmacists give more time and attention to their patients than physicians do.

I suppose one could make the argument that at this time of HMOs, it's not easy for physicians to spend enough time with their patients. For those of people I have just a few words to say: It is not easy for pharmacists, either. Being a community pharmacist I can assure you that we run like a machine, all day long. Even machines are better off than we are, since the attending person will turn the machine off once and a while to give it a rest, while we pharmacists often have no time to even go to the restroom.

One additional factor plays a role in making up this quote and gave pharmacists the highest ranking in this area for such a long time. That is, simply, the easy access for anyone and the availability of the pharmacist to answer questions and clarify concerns that patients might have.

Now to go back to the earlier question: Why doesn't the general public respect pharmacists?

As I said before, I was unsuccessful in finding an answer, but I think one of the reasons—not the whole reason—is the concept of "customer service," which has been implanted in people's minds. The idea that "customer first," might apply to certain fields of business; but, sorry, it is not exactly valid for, the pharmacy business.

I'm not sure what percentage of pharmacists feel this way, but at the end of the day, the matter that bothers me the most and even haunts me on a personal level, is the treatment I face when dealing with patients, when disrespect manifests itself clearly, whether directly or indirectly.

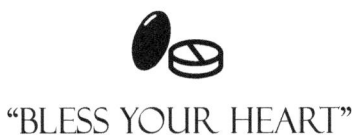

"BLESS YOUR HEART"

One issue that any community pharmacist deals with many times on any given day is counseling patients. Among these counseling scenarios, the pharmacist will face the necessity to warn a tremendous number of patients about the side effects of certain medications, especially controlled medicines. We have to explain possible drowsiness, the need to be careful about interactions between drugs, the potential for addiction, and substances the patient should avoid while taking this medicine.

Any pharmacist knows these facts as well as we know that 2+2=4. But sometimes, we face situations in which we are caught between anger and laughter.

As we all agree, there is no such thing as a stupid question, taking into consideration that not everybody who takes medicine has all the necessary knowledge and details about it. However, some of the questions patients ask are just outrageous, if not ridiculous.

I received a phone call from a patient who asked whether adding an alcoholic beverage to the formula of Vicodin and Soma that he was taking for a back injury would maximize the pain relief. According to him, a friend of his wife gave him this piece of advice! (I wonder how often advice like this is applied without consulting health care professionals – and how severe the damage is.)

Of course, I had to be professional in my answer. I advised him that this was not a good idea, explained the reasoning behind my advice, and gave enough warning in this case.

I think having the community pharmacy around the corner, with a pharmacist available around the clock, is one of the nicest things any community can have. Imagine that you are cooking a new recipe, and you are stuck in the middle with one question. You wonder whom you can call and ask (especially when you're looking for a professional answer, not your next-door neighbor's help).

Well, people, please allow me to say, humbly, bless your pharmacist's heart, he or she is there for you.

"KEEP AN EYE ON THE SUPPLY."

No one can disagree with the idea that a large part of the profession of pharmacy consists of dealing with the human side of every prescription that the pharmacist fills, regardless of whom it is for or what reason it is filled for.

We all deal on a daily basis with one human interaction or another. Even when you take your car to the mechanic, there is an interaction. But with a community pharmacy, this relation is much more emphasized, with extra details, since it touches an important part of life, and that is health.

I try always to be professional without forgetting the human touch we will seek in our interactions with others. I do my best to remind myself that it's important to fill every prescription correctly and efficiently, but at the same time it is crucial to add that human touch when approaching the patient, who usually expects the right doctor's order to be delivered with an easy to access and with a friendly approach.

The pharmacist, in my opinion, has to be professional with a sympathetic tone. This brings us to the second area of interaction with patients, which is simply the lines that the pharmacist has to draw to avoid giving the impression that it's OK to use and abuse the relationship with the pharmacist.

This is a critical issue, and it's not an easy process to draw those lines, since they are fine and vague in certain situations. In other words, the pharmacist has to be professional, showing sympathy toward the patient without being too open or super friendly.

It could be me personally or the normal thing to believe everything that a person might tell you. I'm one of those people who believe almost everything other people say. So, I react to any given situation based purely on what I hear, without passing it first through a lie detector or a mesh of truth. My explanation is that I'm neither a policewoman nor a judge in a courthouse, and I know only one thing: There is a fact or a problem, followed by a process of interaction between the pharmacist and the patient which ultimately will take us to a resolution.

Knowing all the facts in the previous introduction, I can now relate an incident that happened to me and forced me, as a result, to bring up the issue as a whole.

A regular patient at the location where I work has a history of pain medication for which we fill his prescriptions on a regular basis. His file shows all kinds of situations, including a worker's compensation case, a history of back injuries, a car accident, chronic headache pain, and so on. The pharmacists here tried to do their jobs by always counseling the patient about the dangers of abusing these kinds of medicine and their habit-forming properties, and by contacting the doctors prescribing these drugs to make sure that everything is clear to them before prescribing and later on dispensing these drugs. When the prescribing doctors are convinced and the orders for these medications are clear and necessary, the pharmacist will usually fill them without a second thought.

One day, this patient stepped into the pharmacy and handed me a prescription with a list of medications. While I was typing the list, he started telling me that he had had a heart attack a few days earlier. My reaction was to sympathize with him and show my sincere concern.

The following week, a pharmacy colleague told me that the same patient had approached her recently with a prescription order (actually a list of medications) to prepare him for an upcoming surgical procedure. She said that he handed her the prescription with a delighted attitude, just the opposite of what you would expect from a person who was scheduled for surgery in the upcoming days.

When I told her how sorry I had been to hear about his recent heart attack, she was surprised, since she had dealt with this patient more often than I had and knew that his scenario of life is a sequence of events that will never stop, through which he makes sure that he will never even come close to running out of pain medication.

I felt bad for two reasons. First, I was sorry for sympathizing with somebody who was basically using me and the pharmacy to meet his needs. Second, this patient is focused, not on enjoying life, but on providing himself and his abusive habit with an endless supply of pain medication.

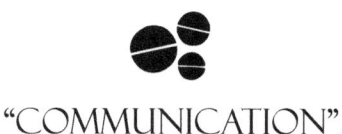

"COMMUNICATION"

When I decided to start working on this book, one of the main things on my mind was that it had to be of value, or had to give at least a certain amount of benefit, to all pharmacy school students, specifically those who were considering a future in community pharmacy.

Almost all schools today have some classes in public speaking, which will prepare the student for real-life matters. Well, in pharmacy schools I think this is a very important area where schools have to give and spend a great deal of time and effort in implanting that in their students.

I'm talking about anything that has to do with communication, interpersonal interactions, and human relationships in general. These aspects are as important as the science and information that students work hard to achieve a good grade in.

With my experience in community pharmacy, I can say easily and with great confidence that the kind of communication between the pharmacist and the patient plays a big role in the outcome of the patient's medical treatment—the reason the patient came to the pharmacy in the first place.

Even though my explanation of the instructions will not be the sole reason for a good result from taking the medicine, I believe strongly that this accounts for at least one-third of the responsibility that any case of a given patient is when it comes to therapy and medicines.

Therefore, when the pharmacist has a good background in that area, the patient's cumulative experience from everyday interactions will strengthen their relationship, and the ultimate result will be a great benefit to that specific patient's treatment protocol.

Communication typically involves a range of issues, from minor things to very important matters. It starts with the way the pharmacist dresses and includes the pharmacist's approach to the patient with a simple word like "Hi"; the smile on the pharmacist's face; and the tone and volume of his or her voice.

I approach each patient with the intention of offering my best to him or her, whether it is a piece of information or a concern in mind. I have found that this attitude always pays off very well, even with a patient who has problems with the world in general. That patient will carry this kind of attitude whether he or she goes to a restaurant, talks with a bank agent, or, in this case, comes to the pharmacy to fill a prescription!

At the beginning of my practice as a pharmacist, it used to hurt me a lot when a patient would act or react badly when I tried to offer my help or answer questions. Negative attitudes and reactions don't affect me anymore. The reason for that might be simply because I start looking at the whole subject from a completely different aspect since it's the patient's problem and not mine.

Again, I think the way you smile and greet your patient makes up almost one-third of the whole interaction or counseling you practice every day as a community pharmacist. When you add to that good knowledge, a big heart, and an open mind for the simplest human needs, then, believe me, this recipe will produce a great pharmacist who can and will serve his or her community and go home with an excellent degree of satisfaction from this profession.

"YOU'VE GOT A QUESTION... I'VE GOT AN ANSWER."

Sometimes, it's really funny how a patient asks a question, and then, in less than a week, they will repeat the same question, even though you thought that your answer was clear and to the point!

I had a patient who wondered what the difference was between two medications, Soma (Carisoprodol) and Flexeril (Cyclobenzaprine).

These two muscle relaxants are very popular, as you might know, and there is a certain degree of dependency or habit forming with them. I guess that when I answered the patient the first time, there was a different question behind this straightforward question.

I later found out that this patient had taken Soma for a while, and had apparently abused it. When her doctor decided to switch her to Flexeril, she wasn't happy with that.

As I said before, even though these two medications might be used for the same indication, it appears that Soma is more popular and is abused more frequently.

When the patient started on Flexeril, she expected the same result that she used to have while taking Soma, but that scenario didn't occur.

Now the patient was doubly angry because her doctor had made the switch, and because she was unhappy with the outcome of taking Flexeril.

Obviously, when I answered her question, I didn't give the answer she was expecting, since she didn't ask me the real question she was wondering about in the first place. While I feel sorry for the whole situation that the patient has to deal with, I think the doctor and the pharmacist can and will play a tremendous role in these cases.

When the doctor makes a change in the person's protocol of medicine, he or she has to explain the reason for the change. Then comes the pharmacist's role. When a patient approaches him or her with a clearly expressed concern, then he or she can explain the matter in a more direct way.

"WHAT FLAVOR WOULD YOU LIKE FOR YOUR ANTIDEPRESSANT DRINK?"

Even though depression has been known as a medical condition for a long time, it's really got you by surprise how widespread this condition is.

We might understand the fact that depression affects a certain percentage of people, which also could take them to the next step of seeing a physician and filling a prescription for an antidepressant, yet it's hard to explain how society has ended up with a near epidemic of depression!

Times change, and people change. New things happen; after a while, these become the norm and not the exception. Old things might vanish, and people forget completely about them.

Being a community pharmacist puts you in a situation that is unique in many different aspects. One of those aspects is dealing with antidepressant medications every day. It makes you ask: Is it true that there are that many depressed people out there?

Since I don't have statistics or a scientific study in front of me, I can't just jump to conclusions or assume a situation. However, I can certainly say that most of the antidepressant prescriptions we handle in the pharmacy every day are more like mood elevators than antidepressants.

Unfortunately, it has begun to seem abnormal and strange to meet somebody who is not taking any kind of antidepressant! I remember hearing a conversation between two high school students in which one of them was upset and angry at her physician because he refused to give her one of the antidepressant medications she had asked for. Of course,

I didn't tell that person this, but the reason this physician declined her request is simply because she didn't have a condition that required such a treatment. But obviously, she thought otherwise.

While I hate to be negative in my approach, I can see, maybe twenty years or less clown the road, that we will be able to buy an over-the-counter preparation, whether in a tablet form or as a drink, which has an antidepressant as its base. So just imagine, instead of getting a bottle of juice or coffee or one of those multivitamin drinks, you will get a drink of antidepressant. And as much as I don't wish for this to happen, I have a strong feeling that this scenario will not stay as a scenario, but will become a normal thing, just other trends that will become a part of everyday life.

"SORRY... I DON'T NEED TO SEE THE SPECIMEN."

When I started working on this book, my intention was not to tell weird or strange stories that had happened to me, or that I had heard of while working in the pharmacy. With my apology, though, this is that kind of story.

An elderly patient stopped by the pharmacy and requested a pharmacist's help. It happened to be my luck to help him. He stated his request, and for a moment I thought I misunderstood him or wasn't following him correctly. Indeed, neither was right, and the question is clear and right to the point; but, are you ready to know what it was?

The patient, or the caretaker, put on the container at the counseling table. It was a small Ziploc bag (like one you would use for snacks or a sandwich), and in that bag was a small thing, about one-half inch in size, brown in color, and semi-solid in consistency.

He opened his hand to show me three different kinds of medicine—two tablets and one capsule—that I was familiar with, and said that he was wondering if any of these medicines would end up in his bowel movements; for example, the sample he kept in the Ziploc bag. In other words, he was asking me if this sample bowel movement contained any of these medicines.

While we pharmacists do, indeed, study the pharmodynamic and the pharmokinetic effects of almost every medicine, we don't really know what they end up as in the bowel movement.

Despite the severe case of nausea I felt then, since I usually don't deal with specimens or any kind of human product or fluid, I tried to pull myself together and explain to that patient, in an honest and professional way, that I have no idea what that specimen held, if anything, or what any of those medicines he had in his hand usually look like in a bowel movement.

I did explain to him that there are very few medicines that do retain a distinctive shape or form in the bowel movement and that his medicines were not in this group.

That elderly person left the pharmacy unhappy, mumbling about how disappointed he was, clearly by talking to his wife who was standing next to him. Obviously, he was expecting that I should know the answer, easily and quickly.

I followed him with my eyes as he left the pharmacy. I was speechless and astonished. Most important, I was disgusted, since I thought the whole situation from the beginning was so weird.

I can completely understand his concern, and I agree that he might have some questions about the specimen he carried in the lovely Ziploc bag, but I cannot believe or imagine that such a thing could face a pharmacist in a community pharmacy. I just wish he had approached me with the question without the bowel movement specimen since this did not help in solving the mystery. Actually, all it accomplished was to cause me not to have my lunch that day, and I know for sure that you don't blame me for that.

"A HOLIDAY WITH TEARS."

I know that the subject of people's attitudes during the holidays has been on the table before. There is always something new to add, though, since it's a subject with different views and aspects.

The place is a community pharmacy, the time is a Sunday exactly two weeks before New Year's Day, and the actual scenario is simply a patient with a prescription for antidepressant medicine. So, where is the problem? It is basically another challenging issue with an insurance company.

The previous Friday, the patient had stopped by the pharmacy to fill her prescription. Unfortunately, her insurance company had declined her prescription for ninety tablets (in this case, a month's supply). That Friday happened to be my day off. According to the patient, the pharmacy had informed her that her insurance company required prior authorization (which is a special procedure that usually involves the patient's insurance company and his or her physician to ensure that certain medicines that are not usually covered will be covered in a particular situation).

Now, let's get to the real facts (and forget all scenarios!). That day, I faced a patient in a rage and full of anger who wants her medicine ready at that moment, without any concern about what had happened on Friday which I thought she fully understood.

The funny—or maybe sad—part is how angry she became when I first tried to find out what was going on with that prescription. Since I had not been at work that day, I started to research the case, as we usually do in such situations.

I really would love to have a video camera that can catch what's going on, both in sound and picture, as I tried to research the situation while the patient fired on me and on the pharmacy all the questions and the unacceptable matter: How come her medicine was not ready?

I was lucky to find out what was going on. I found the paperwork attached to the prescription. It stated that a prior authorization request had been faxed from our pharmacy to the patient's insurance company on Friday afternoon.

I quickly brought the paperwork to the patient and started explaining to her why her medicine was not ready to be picked up. There is no fixed time for any prior authorization request, but by simple calculation, since it was requested on Friday afternoon and usually takes, on average, three days to approve such a request, it would be impossible to have the medicine ready on Sun-day afternoon (unless, of course, she wanted to pay for part or all of the prescription herself).

When this story started, the patient was 95 percent mad and angry. Now had reached 150 percent plus. She was convinced that it was the pharmacy's fault and nobody else's. If the pharmacy was efficient enough, she thought, this would not have happened. I tried to calm her down by offering her a few tablets with no charge until her prescription was approved by her insurance company and suggesting that, if she preferred, she could have the prescription filled completely by paying for it out of pocket; if it was approved later she would be reimbursed. Unfortunately, all of my efforts were worthless.

At that moment she screamed, "Get me a manager." It was Sun-day, and he was at home enjoying the weekend. When I explained this, she rushed to the store manager (I work in a retail setting).

A few moments later, I saw her leaving the store. Then the store manager approached me to inquire about the issue. I explained briefly what had happened, and he stated that he was unable to pinpoint the problem. The only thing he was sure about was how angry and agitated the patient was. He had seen her leave the store and stand outside, crying.

After all, regardless of the details, I don't want any patient leaving the pharmacy in tears. 1 repeated the scenario in my head and tried to locate any mishandling from the pharmacy's side, but clearly there were none. The only explanation I could find was, again, holiday stress.

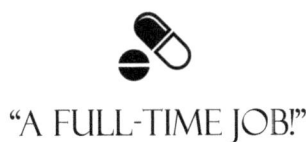

"A FULL-TIME JOB!"

Question: How would you feel if someone at your job was doing something illegal or unethical, making you a middleman or woman for that act? Of course, let me make this clear, you wouldn't have any idea that you were playing a key role in this ugly and unacceptable game!

Before I go into the specific details, 1 have to admit that I honestly don't know whether the case I'm dealing with is separate and isolated or a more common and popular case, a real problem our society suffers silently from. It is difficult to tell because of the limited data and information available to the public from an authorized and dependable source.

This real-life scenario happened at the community pharmacy where I work. A patient filled his prescription for a painkiller called "Norco," a combination of hydrocodone and acetaminophen. One day later, he came by with other painkillers, much stronger this time, called OxyContin, a delayed-release form of oxycodone.

My first reaction was to give the benefit of the doubt to the patient and his condition. I assumed that Norco had not done the job as far as taking care of the pain went, and he might have needed something like Oxycontin for more severe pain. But there was a red flag: The second prescription was from a different doctor's office. So the pharmacy called the second doctor to verify that he was aware that the patient was already on Norco.

It took just a few minutes to verify that, and the doctor requested that the pharmacist withhold the prescription for Oxycontin until he could reach the doctor who had prescribed Norco originally.

Of course, our patient wasn't happy at all about this. He left the pharmacy angry and swearing at the pharmacy and its staff.

After two days, I received a phone call, this time from the doctor who had prescribed Norco. Almost 100 percent of this physician's prescriptions are for painkillers since he is a pain management specialist. He told me that he had performed a urine test for that patient and found it 100 percent clean of any kind of painkiller ingredients. His conclusion was that the patient had not taken any of the Norco that he had originally prescribed, and he did not know why the patient had gone to the other physician to obtain another prescription for even stronger pain medication.

Maybe out of curiosity, or because 1 really wanted to know this doctor's position on this case, I asked him if he was going to keep the patient as one of his clients, and to my surprise, he said, "Yes, I will."

A few hours later, a call came from the second physician, who wasn't a pain management specialist. He informed me that he had spoken to the specialist and was told the same information 1 had received from him earlier that day. The only new pieces of information this time were that the second physician wanted me to discard the prescription completely and that he would not welcome that patient into his office in the future.

At this point, it might be very clear that there is only one logical explanation for this story. You have a patient going to different physicians' offices, looking for a prescription for pain medicine. Since he is obviously not taking any of them, what he is really doing with all of them?

That takes us to the beginning of this article, about being used by somebody else to obtain or perform an illegal or unethical act. This patient simply used me and my pharmacy for his unacceptable activities. He was lucky until a small red flag appeared in the way and stopped his mission.

I just wonder how many times he was successful in achieving his goal. I even wonder if this is his full-time job!